THE
HEALING
PLATE

Optimizing Nutrition for Living with HIV/AIDS

Dr Macklene.C. Jones

CONTENTS

Introduction

Living with HIV/AIDS brings unique challenges, and one of the most important factors to consider for people living with this disease is diet. A well-balanced, nutrient-dense diet is critical for immune system support, symptom management, and general well-being. This book is intended to be a comprehensive resource for anyone looking to improve their nutrition and make informed decisions to improve their health while living with HIV/AIDS.

In this book, we will look at the relationship between HIV/AIDS and nutrition, how the infection impacts the body's nutritional demands, and how to overcome typical obstacles. We will look at the essential nutrients needed for immune support and how to create a well-rounded food plan that includes these elements in a practical and enjoyable approach. We will also talk about portion control, mindful eating, and the necessity of hydration for people living with HIV/AIDS.

This book is all about being practical. We will supply you with a plethora of information and resources to assist you in putting the principles presented into practice. We hope to empower you to make informed decisions and take control of your health journey by providing a thorough list of nutrient-rich foods as well as practical meal preparation recommendations.

It is crucial to emphasize that this book is not intended to replace expert medical advice. It should be used in conjunction with advice from your healthcare professional, who may make tailored suggestions based on your unique needs and medical condition.

By utilizing the knowledge and tactics provided with the information in this book, you will be able to optimize your diet and improve your general well-being while living with HIV/AIDS. Let's go on this adventure together to nourish and nurture your body, allowing you to live a healthy and fulfilling life.

Chapter 1

Recognizing HIV/AIDS and Its Impact on Nutrition

Living with HIV/AIDS poses unique problems, not just in terms of physical health, but also in terms of diet. In this chapter, we will look at the basics of HIV/AIDS, including its impact on the body's nutritional demands and the critical role nutrition plays in managing the condition.

1.1 What exactly is HIV/AIDS?

- HIV (Human Immunodeficiency Virus) and AIDS (acquired immunodeficiency syndrome) Overview
- The disease's transmission, stages, and progression
- HIV/AIDS prevalence and global influence

1.2 The HIV/AIDS and Nutrition Connection

- The impact of HIV on the immune system and metabolic systems
- HIV's effect on nutritional uptake and utilization
- Common nutritional deficits and their effects in HIV/AIDS patients

1.3 Nutritional Difficulties in HIV/AIDS

Factors that contribute to malnutrition in HIV/AIDS patients

- Appetite and food consumption changes
- Complications in the gastrointestinal tract and problems with nutrition absorption
- The effect of opportunistic infections on nutrition

1.4 Immune Function and Nutrition's Role

- The significance of a healthy immune system in HIV/AIDS management
- Nutritional effects on immunological function
- Key immune-boosting nutrients and their sources

1.5 Medical Aspects of HIV/AIDS Nutrition

Antiretroviral treatment (ART) and diet interactions

- Medication side effects and their impact on dietary choices
- Considering drug-nutrient interactions and possible consequences

1.6 Seeking Professional Advice

- The role of healthcare practitioners in HIV/AIDS nutrition management
- The significance of multidisciplinary care teams
- Locating a licensed dietitian or nutritionist with HIV/AIDS competence

Individuals living with HIV/AIDS must understand the intricate interaction between HIV/AIDS and nutrition. We may begin to establish methods to address and overcome obstacles by understanding the impact of HIV/AIDS on the body's nutritional needs and recognizing the challenges that may occur. In the next chapters, we will look at how to create a nutritious and nourishing diet that supports immune function and overall well-being for people living with HIV/AIDS.

1.1 What Exactly is HIV/AIDS?

HIV (Human Immunodeficiency Virus) is a virus that assaults the immune system, primarily CD4 cells, a type of white blood cell that is essential for battling infections and disorders. If HIV is not treated, it can progress to AIDS (acquired immunodeficiency syndrome).

HIV is primarily spread by bodily fluids such as blood, sperm, vaginal secretions, and breast milk. Unprotected sexual contact, sharing contaminated needles or syringes, mother-to-child transmission during childbirth or breastfeeding, and, less commonly, blood transfusions (though this is rare in many countries where blood donations are screened for HIV) are the most common modes of transmission.

When the virus enters the body, it gradually weakens the immune system, rendering people more vulnerable to opportunistic infections as well as certain types of cancer. When a person with HIV suffers from severe immune system damage, such as a significantly low CD4 cell count or the emergence of particular opportunistic infections or malignancies, AIDS is diagnosed.

Although there is no cure for HIV/AIDS at the moment, considerable advances in treatment and care have been accomplished. The conventional treatment for HIV/AIDS is antiretroviral therapy (ART), which consists of a mix of drugs that help suppress the virus, protect immunological function, and improve overall health outcomes. People living with HIV can live long and healthy lives with good medical care and commitment to therapy.

It is critical to understand that HIV is not spread by casual contact such as hugging, shaking hands, or sharing food or drinks. Learning more about HIV/AIDS prevention, safe behavior, and increasing knowledge and compassion are critical in preventing new infections and reducing the condition's stigma.

1.2 The HIV/AIDS and Nutrition Connection

The link between HIV/AIDS and diet is complex and diverse. HIV/AIDS can have a substantial impact on the body's nutritional requirements, and good nutrition is critical in controlling the condition and sustaining general health. Here are some essential characteristics of the HIV/AIDS-nutrition relationship:

1.2.1 Impaired Nutrient Absorption and Utilization: HIV can damage the body's ability to effectively absorb and utilize nutrients. The virus can induce inflammation and damage to the gastrointestinal tract, resulting in nutrient loss. Even if an individual's dietary intake is adequate, this can result in nutrient shortages. Vitamins (such as B12, D, and folate), minerals (such as iron, zinc, and selenium), and macronutrients (such as proteins, carbs, and fats) are commonly affected.

1.2.2 Increased Nutritional Needs: Living with HIV/AIDS raises the body's nutritional needs. To combat the infection, the immune system requires additional energy and nutrition. Increased metabolic demands, combined with nutritional absorption and utilization problems, can contribute to malnutrition and weight loss in HIV/AIDS patients.

1.2.3 Immune System Weakness: HIV/AIDS affects the immune system, making people more susceptible to infections and opportunistic illnesses. An adequate diet is critical for immune function and the body's ability to fight infections. Nutrients like Vitamin C, vitamin A, zinc, selenium, and omega-3 fatty acids all play important roles in immune response enhancement.

1.2.4 The Influence of Opportunistic Infections:

Opportunistic infections, or infections that take advantage of a weakened immune system, are common in HIV/AIDS patients. These infections can have an impact on nutritional status by reducing appetite, promoting nutrient malabsorption, and increasing nutrient requirements. Conditions such as oral thrush or esophagitis, for example, can make eating and swallowing uncomfortable, resulting in decreased food intake and potential nutrient deficits.

1.2.5 Adverse Antiretroviral Therapy (ART) Effects:

While antiretroviral therapy (ART) is necessary for HIV/AIDS management, it can have nutritional adverse effects. Some drugs can produce gastrointestinal problems, changed taste perception, or changes in fat metabolism, all of which can have an impact on dietary intake and nutrient absorption. While on ART, it is critical to control these adverse effects and collaborate with healthcare experts to maintain proper nutrition.

Understanding the link between HIV/AIDS and nutrition is critical for designing strategies to improve nutritional status and overall health. In the next chapters, we will look at how to design a nutritious and nourishing diet, how to address the specific nutritional issues that people living with HIV/AIDS encounter, and how to promote optimal well-being in the face of this condition.

1.3 Nutritional Issues in HIV/AIDS

Individuals living with HIV/AIDS confront several nutritional problems that can have a negative influence on their general health and well-being. These difficulties develop as a result of the complicated interactions between the virus, the immune system, and the metabolic processes of the body. Here are some of the most common nutritional difficulties with HIV/AIDS:

1.3.1 Increased Nutritional Needs: HIV/AIDS raises the body's nutritional needs due to variables such as chronic inflammation, raised metabolic rate, and increased energy and nutrient demands of the immune system. Meeting these additional demands might be difficult, especially if food absorption or appetite is impaired.

1.3.2 Malnutrition and Weight Loss: Malnutrition is a major problem in HIV/AIDS patients. The virus can affect nutrient absorption, and nutrient utilization, and lead to disease, diminished appetite, or changed taste sensations. As a result, weight loss and muscle wasting can occur, compromising nutritional status and increasing susceptibility to infections and other problems.

1.3.3 Micronutrient Deficiencies: People living with HIV/AIDS may be deficient in certain vitamins and minerals. Malabsorption, increased nutrient use, and decreased intake can all contribute to nutrient deficits in vitamins B12, D, folate, iron, zinc, and selenium. These inadequacies can weaken the immune system even further, impede recovery, and have a severe influence on overall health.

1.3.4 Gastrointestinal Problems: HIV/AIDS can impact the gastrointestinal tract, causing a variety of digestive problems. Diarrhea, malabsorption, nausea, vomiting, and mouth or throat sores are all common gastrointestinal problems. These issues can impede food absorption and consumption, worsening nutritional difficulties and contributing to weight loss and malnutrition.

1.3.5 Medication Side Effects: While antiretroviral therapy (ART) is essential in the treatment of HIV/AIDS, it can have nutritional adverse effects. Some drugs may cause gastrointestinal problems, changes in taste perception, or changes in fat metabolism. These side effects can impair appetite, food absorption, and utilization, making proper nutrition more difficult to achieve.

1.3.6 Psychological and Social Factors: Psychological and social factors can also play a role in HIV/AIDS nutritional problems. Depression, stigma, a lack of healthful food options, and socioeconomic issues can all have an impact on dietary choices, food security, and general nutrition.

To address these nutritional difficulties, a multifaceted approach that combines medical management, dietary interventions, and psychological support is required. Working with a healthcare team that includes an HIV/AIDS licensed dietitian or nutritionist might be beneficial. Individuals create tailored nutrition plans to fulfill their specific nutritional demands, maximize nutrient consumption, and promote overall health and well-being.

1.4 Immune Function and Nutrition's Role

The immune system is critical in the treatment of HIV/AIDS. The immune system protects the body from infections, illnesses, and other potentially dangerous chemicals. Proper nutrition is critical for immune function and maximizing the body's ability to fight HIV and its consequences. Here are some crucial points about immune function and the importance of diet in HIV/AIDS:

1.4.1 The Importance of a Healthy Immune System: Individuals living with HIV/AIDS require a strong immune system. It aids in the regulation of viral replication, the suppression of opportunistic infections, and the maintenance of overall health. HIV, on the other hand, assaults and gradually weakens the immune system, making people more vulnerable to infections and illnesses. Nutritional support for immune function is critical for improving outcomes and overall well-being.

1.4.2 Immune Supporting Nutrients:

Certain nutrients are essential for immunological function.

These are some examples:
- Protein is required for the formation of antibodies and immune cells.

- Vitamins: Vitamins A, C, E, and D all have roles in immunological processes such as antibody formation, cellular immunity, and antioxidant protection.
- Minerals such as zinc, selenium, iron, and copper help immune cells function and antioxidant defenses.
- Omega-3 fatty acids: Found in fish, flaxseeds, and chia seeds, they have anti-inflammatory qualities and help regulate the immune system.
- Antioxidants: Antioxidants, which are found in fruits, vegetables, and whole grains, aid in minimizing oxidative stress and boost immunological health.

1.4.3 Malnutrition's Influence on Immune Function: Malnutrition is a condition in which Immune function is compromised in those living with HIV/AIDS. Inadequate nutritional intake inhibits immune cell development and function, lowers antibody response, and weakens the body's ability to fight infections. Malnutrition can make you more susceptible to opportunistic infections and make you recover from illnesses more slowly.

1.4.4 Immune Support Nutritional Strategies:

Nutritional optimization can aid immune function in people living with HIV/AIDS.

Among the key strategies are:

- Maintaining a healthy diet: Fruits, vegetables, whole grains, lean meats, and healthy fats should be prioritized.
- Meeting increased protein and energy requirements: Adequate calorie and protein intake is critical for immunological function and muscle preservation.
- Taking care of certain vitamin deficiencies: Work with a healthcare physician or certified dietitian to diagnose and correct vitamin, mineral, and nutrient deficiencies.
- Promoting Gut Health: The gut is an important part of the immune system. Probiotic-rich meals and prebiotic fiber can help maintain a healthy gut flora and improve immune function.

- Keeping hydrated: Staying hydrated promotes optimum immune responses and general health.

1.4.5 Antiretroviral Therapy (ART) Interactions:

Nutrition can alter the effectiveness and negative effects of antiretroviral therapy (ART). Some nutrients may interfere with the absorption or efficacy of ART drugs. It is critical to collaborate closely with healthcare experts to ensure optimal timing and potential drug and nutritional strategy modifications.

Individuals with HIV/AIDS can improve their overall health outcomes and better control their condition by prioritizing diet and immunological function. A well-planned and balanced diet, as well as proper medical care, can play a significant role in supporting the immune system and overall wellbeing

1.5 Medical Aspects of HIV/AIDS Nutrition

Individuals living with HIV/AIDS require a proper diet to sustain their overall health and well-being. When addressing nutrition in the context of HIV/AIDS, various medical factors must be taken into account. Among these factors are:

1.5.1 Antiretroviral Therapy (ART) Interactions:

The cornerstone of HIV/AIDS treatment is antiretroviral therapy (ART). It aids in the suppression of viral replication, the preservation of immune function, and the improvement of overall health outcomes. In terms of nutrition, several ART drugs can interact with meals, reducing absorption or effectiveness. It is critical to follow the particular advice offered by healthcare experts regarding food and medication interactions. Some prescriptions must be taken with or without food, while certain foods or supplements must be taken with or without food. To avoid harmful interactions, some foods or supplements may need to be avoided.

1.5.2 Medication Side Effects:

Antiretroviral medicines used in HIV/AIDS treatment might have nutritional adverse effects. Gestural abnormalities, changed taste perception, alterations in lipid metabolism, and bone health concerns are all typical side effects. These side effects have the potential to impair appetite, nutritional absorption, and overall dietary intake. Working together with healthcare practitioners and licensed dietitians/nutritionists can aid in the management of these side effects and the implementation of essential dietary changes to ensure adequate nutrition.

1.5.3 Handling Gastrointestinal Complaints:

Individuals living with HIV/AIDS may suffer from gastrointestinal symptoms such as diarrhea, nausea, vomiting, and mouth sores, which can interfere with nutritional intake and nutrient absorption. It is critical to address these symptoms to prevent malnutrition and enhance overall health. Avoiding spicy or irritating foods, eating small and frequent meals, staying hydrated, and including easily digestible foods can all help manage gastrointestinal discomfort and increase nutrient intake.

1.5.4 Opportunistic Infection Nutritional Support: Opportunistic infections, which can develop in people with weakened immune systems, may necessitate special dietary considerations. Individuals suffering from oral thrush, for example, may benefit from an anti-inflammatory and antifungal diet, whereas those suffering from malabsorption may require nutrient-dense meals and supplementation to correct deficiencies. Nutritional interventions should be adapted to meet the unique needs and problems of opportunistic illnesses.

1.5.5 Personalized Nutrition Plans:

Individuals with HIV/AIDS may have different dietary demands depending on their age, gender, weight, activity level, and disease progression. Working with healthcare practitioners and licensed dietitians/nutritionists to create tailored nutrition regimens that suit specific needs and goals is critical. These experts can advise you on calorie and macronutrient requirements, optimal nutrient intake, and tracking your progress over time.

1.5.6 Nutritional Status Monitoring:

In HIV/AIDS patients, nutritional status must be monitored regularly. Body weight, body composition, nutrient levels, and laboratory markers of nutritional status may all be evaluated. Monitoring assists in identifying any deficits, changes in nutritional requirements, or pharmaceutical adverse effects that may necessitate changes to the nutrition plan.

Individuals with HIV/AIDS can build tailored dietary regimens that meet their particular needs, increase overall health, and improve disease management by taking these medical considerations into account and working together with healthcare practitioners.

1.6 Seeking Professional Advice

When it comes to nutrition for people living with HIV/AIDS, seeking professional advice is critical. Healthcare practitioners' experience and support, particularly registered dietitians/nutritionists, can greatly contribute to optimizing nutritional intake, managing medical concerns, and increasing general well-being. Here are some of the most essential reasons to seek professional advice:

1.6.1 Individualized Nutrition Evaluation:

Registered dietitians/nutritionists, in particular, can undertake a complete examination of an individual's nutritional needs, medical history, and specific goals. This evaluation considers characteristics such as age, gender, weight, disease progression, medication regimen, and any pre-existing medical problems. It permits the creation of a personalized nutrition plan that is suited to the individual's specific needs.

1.6.2 Appropriate Nutrient Intake:

Professionals can advise you on how to get the most out of your nutrient consumption in line with the increased nutritional needs of patients with HIV/AIDS. They can assist in the identification of potential nutrient deficiencies, the development of strategies to address them, and the recommendation of specific food sources or supplements to guarantee appropriate consumption of vital vitamins, minerals, and macronutrients.

1.6.3 Management of Medication and Nutritional Interactions:

Antiretroviral therapy (ART) is an important part of HIV/AIDS treatment, and healthcare providers are well-versed in pharmaceutical and dietary interactions. They can advise on medication delivery scheduling about meals, nutrient depletion induced by medications, and the avoidance of specific foods or supplements that may interfere with medication effectiveness.

1.6.4 Addressing Specific Medical Issues:

Healthcare practitioners are prepared to address the medical concerns related to HIV/AIDS nutrition. They can aid in the management of side effects. Medication side effects can include impaired taste perception, gastrointestinal difficulties, and bone health issues. They can provide advice on how to manage symptoms associated with opportunistic infections, as well as how to ensure sufficient nutrition during periods of illness or decreased gastrointestinal function

1.6.5 Monitoring and Adjustments:

Regular nutritional status monitoring is required to assess progress and make any changes to the nutrition plan. Healthcare providers can monitor changes in body weight, body composition, and nutrient levels, as well as any changes in nutritional requirements or drug regimes. This constant monitoring enables changes to the dietary plan to be made as needed to optimize results.

1.6.6 Emotional and Psychosocial Assistance:

In addition to nutritional advice, healthcare providers can provide emotional and psychosocial support to people living with

HIV/AIDS. They can address concerns about body image issues, dietary problems, stigma, and other psychosocial factors that can all have an impact on nutritional well-being. This all-encompassing approach assists people in navigating the emotional components of their condition and developing a positive relationship with food and nutrition.

It is important to remember that healthcare providers, especially registered dietitians/nutritionists, are important members of the healthcare team. They have specialist expertise and experience in HIV/AIDS nutrition and can provide advice customized to each individual's specific needs and circumstances. By enlisting their help, you can guarantee that your nutrition programs are evidence-based, thorough,

Chapter 2

Essential Nutrients for Immune Support

These nutrients play an important role in building a strong immune system, combating infections, and boosting overall health. Understanding their significance and adding them to a well-balanced diet will improve immune support dramatically. Here are some crucial essential nutrients to discuss:

2.1 Protein: Protein is necessary for immune function since it is involved in the creation of antibodies, cytokines, and immune cells. Protein is required to promote the body's immunological response and recuperation. Lean meats, poultry, fish, eggs, dairy products, legumes, and plant-based proteins are all good sources of protein; Tofu, tempeh, and lentils are examples.

2.2 **Vitamin A**: Vitamin A is involved in a variety of immunological activities, including immune cell formation and function. It aids in the preservation of the integrity of mucosal surfaces, which act as barriers against pathogens. Orange and yellow fruits and vegetables (carrots, sweet potatoes, apricots), leafy green vegetables, liver, and dairy products are all good sources of vitamin A.

2.3 **Vitamin C**: Vitamin C is a potent antioxidant that promotes the development of white blood cells and antibodies, which aids in immune function. It also boosts the activity of natural killer cells, which are critical in the battle against infections. Vitamin C is abundant in citrus

fruits, berries, kiwi, tomatoes, peppers, and leafy green vegetables.

2.4 Vitamin E: Another antioxidant is vitamin E which aids in the protection of immunological cells against oxidative stress. It helps immune cells operate properly and improves the body's reaction to infections. Vitamin E is found in nuts and seeds (almonds, sunflower seeds), vegetable oils, spinach, and broccoli.

2.5 Vitamin D: Vitamin D is essential for immunological modulation and infection resistance. It modulates the immune response, enhances antimicrobial activity, and helps immune cells operate. Sunlight is the best source of vitamin D, although it can also be gotten via fatty fish, fortified dairy products, and pills if necessary.

2.6 Zinc: Zinc is required for the growth and function of immune cells. It aids in the regulation

of immune cell function, increases antibody production, and promotes wound healing. Good zinc sources like Oysters, meat, chicken, beans, almonds, and whole grains are among examples.

2.7 Selenium: Selenium is a mineral that helps the immune system work properly. It is an antioxidant that promotes the activation of certain immune cells. Selenium is found in Brazil nuts, fish, chicken, whole grains, and dairy products.

2.8 Omega-3 Fatty Acids: Omega-3 fatty acids, specifically EPA (eicosatetraenoic acid) and DHA (docosahexaenoic acid), have anti-inflammatory effects and help regulate the immune system. They can aid in the reduction of inflammation, the promotion of immune cell function, and the enhancement of the body's response to infections. Omega-3 fatty acids are abundant in fatty fish (salmon, mackerel, sardines), flaxseeds, chia seeds, and walnuts.

2.9 Antioxidants: Antioxidants, such as those found in fruits, vegetables, and whole grains, aid in the reduction of oxidative stress, and Immune health should be supported. They scavenge free radicals, which can harm immune cells and weaken immunity. Consuming a variety of colored fruits and vegetables ensures a wide spectrum of antioxidants.

Individuals living with HIV/AIDS can help their immune systems fight infections and maintain general health by consuming these vital nutrients in their diet. Working with healthcare practitioners and licensed dietitians/nutritionists to establish individual nutrient needs, correct any specific deficiencies, and develop a well-rounded, nutrient-dense meal plan is critical.

Creating a Balanced Meal Plan.

Creating a balanced meal plan is critical to ensuring that people living with HIV/AIDS obtain appropriate nutrition and immunological support.

Here are some essential measures to consider the following while developing a balanced food plan:

Assess Individual Nutritional preferences: Begin by determining the individual's nutritional requirements based on criteria such as age, gender, weight, activity level, illness progression, and any special dietary preferences or restrictions. A qualified dietitian/nutritionist can undertake this assessment, taking into account the individual's needs.

Include a Wide Range of Food Groups: A well-balanced meal plan should include a variety of food groups to deliver a variety of vital nutrients. These food groupings are as follows:

Fruits and veggies: Include a variety of colorful fruits and vegetables in your diet because they are high in vitamins, minerals, antioxidants, and fiber. To maximize nutrient consumption, include both raw and cooked alternatives.

Whole Grains: Select whole grain alternatives such as Whole wheat bread, brown rice, quinoa, and oats are all good options. They supply complex carbs, fiber, and essential minerals. Include lean protein sources such as poultry, fish, eggs, lentils, tofu, and low-fat dairy products. These supply critical amino acids for immunological activity and tissue repair.

Healthy Fats: Include avocados, almonds, seeds, and olive oil as sources of healthy fats. These include omega-3 fatty acids and promote overall wellness.

Dairy or Dairy Alternatives: To maintain bone health, include low-fat dairy products or dairy alternatives fortified with calcium and vitamin D.

Emphasize Nutrient Density: Choose nutrient-dense foods, which give a high number of nutrients relative to their calorie content. Fruits, vegetables, whole grains, lean meats, and healthy fats are examples of nutrient-dense foods. Avoid or restrict foods that are heavy in added sugars, saturated fats, and processed components.

Consider Portion Sizes: Pay attention to portion sizes to ensure that the meal plan contains an appropriate mix of nutrients and calories. Portion sizes may vary depending on individual needs, thus consulting a qualified dietitian/nutritionist can assist in determining suitable serving sizes for each food group.

Aim for Consistent Meals and Snacks: Encourage consistent eating patterns and avoid skipping meals. Spread out your meals throughout the day to ensure a consistent supply of energy and nutrients. Include healthy snacks between meals if necessary, such as fruits, almonds, yogurt, or whole grain crackers.

Hydration: Include appropriate hydration in your eating plan. Encourage the use of water and other hydrated liquids throughout the day. Staying hydrated benefits both immune function and general health.

Consider Individual Choices and Cultural Factors: When creating a meal plan, consider the individual's dietary choices, cultural background, and culinary traditions. The inclusion of familiar and pleasurable foods increases the likelihood of sticking to the regimen.

Regular Monitoring and Adjustments: Monitor the individual's nutritional status, weight, and overall health regularly. Adjust the meal plan as necessary to reflect changes in nutritional needs, health conditions, or medication regimes.

Working closely with a qualified dietitian/nutritionist to design a personalized and balanced meal plan that addresses the special needs of those living with HIV/AIDS is critical. They can offer advice, assess progress, and make necessary changes to enhance nutrition and immunological function.

Mindful Eating and Portion Control

Portion control and mindful eating are key strategies that can supplement a well-balanced diet and promote healthy eating habits.

Here's an extension of these ideas:

Portion Control: Portion control is the process of controlling the amount of food taken to maintain an optimal calorie intake and nutrient balance. It is critical since even nutritious meals, when consumed in excess, can contribute to weight gain or other health problems.

Here are some ways to practice portion control:

I. **Learn to Estimate Portion Sizes Using Visual Clues:** Learn to estimate portion sizes using visual clues. A meal of protein (such as chicken or fish) should be roughly the size of a deck of cards, while a serving of grains (such as rice or pasta) should be roughly the size of a deck of cards or a tennis ball is around the size of a serving of fat (such as oil or nuts), and a serving of fat (such as almonds) should be about the size of a thumb.

II.   **Examine Food Labels:** Take note of the portion sizes listed on food labels. Compare the serving size to the amount you normally consume and make any necessary adjustments.

III.   **Use Smaller Plates and Bowls:** Use smaller plates and bowls when serving meals. This can provide the appearance of a fuller plate and aid with portion management.

Mindful Eating: Entails eating deliberately and savoring each bite. This allows your brain to detect fullness and satisfaction, limiting overeating. Cut bigger packets of snacks into smaller, single-serving quantities. This prevents thoughtless eating and promotes attentive nibbling.

Mindful Eating is the discipline of eating mindfully, paying attention to the present moment, and being fully aware of the eating experience. It entails paying attention to your body's hunger and fullness cues, as well as the taste, texture, and enjoyment of food.

Here are some guidelines for mindful eating:

I. Eat without Distractions: Avoid using television, phones, or computers while eating. Concentrate entirely on eating and enjoying your food.

II. **Engage Your Senses**: Pay attention to the flavors, aromas, textures, and colors of the food you're consuming. Be fully present in the moment and enjoy the sensory experience.

III. **Chew slowly and thoroughly**: Chew your meal thoroughly. This not only helps digestion but also allows you to completely appreciate the flavor and texture of each bite.

IV.   **Listen to Your Body**: Pay heed to your body's cues of hunger and fullness. Eat when you are physically hungry and quit when you are satisfied.

V.   **Be Non-Judicial**: Avoid categorizing foods as "good" or "bad." Instead, concentrate on sustaining your body with a variety of nutritious foods while allowing yourself to indulge in indulgences in moderation.

VI.   **Gratitude Practice**: Develop a sense of gratitude for the food you eat and the sustenance it provides your body. Appreciate the time and effort that went into its creation.

You may build a healthier relationship with food, improve digestion, and make more informed decisions that support general well-being by including portion control and mindful eating into your meal plan.

Hydration and Its Significance in HIV/AIDS Management

Hydration is essential for HIV/AIDS management and overall health. Here's more on the importance of hydration and its influence on people living with HIV/AIDS:

Maintains Immune Function: Staying hydrated is critical for maintaining a healthy immune system. To function properly, the immune system needs appropriate hydration, which aids in the transfer of immune cells, nutrients, and antibodies throughout the body. This is especially important for people living with HIV/AIDS, whose immune systems may be impaired.

Medication Absorption: Many HIV/AIDS treatments require enough fluids for efficient absorption and effectiveness. Hydration aids in the distribution of drugs throughout the body, enhancing their therapeutic advantages. Proper hydration also aids in the prevention of any pharmaceutical adverse effects.

Nutrient Transport and Absorption: Hydration is vital for transferring and absorbing nutrients. It aids in the transport of nutrients to cells, tissues, and organs, hence assisting in energy production, immunological response, and general nutritional well-being. This is especially significant for people living with HIV/AIDS, who may have higher nutrient requirements due to their disease and drug use

Opportunistic Infection Prevention: Adequate hydration promotes the body's defensive mechanisms against opportunistic infections, which can be a problem for people living with HIV/AIDS. Hydration aids in the preservation of mucous membrane integrity and improves the operation of protective barriers in the respiratory, gastrointestinal, and urine systems.

Improved Gastrointestinal Function: HIV/AIDS can occasionally cause gastrointestinal difficulties like diarrhea or constipation. Proper hydration prevents dehydration and promotes health. Regular bowel motions help to maintain good gastrointestinal function. It also aids in the relief of symptoms and discomfort linked with certain digestive issues.

Improved Kidney Function: Maintaining normal kidney function requires adequate hydration. It aids in the removal of waste and toxins from the body, lowering the risk of kidney-related problems. Adequate hydration can also help prevent kidney stones, which are more common in HIV/AIDS patients due to particular drugs or metabolic abnormalities.

Overall Health and Energy Levels: Hydration adds to general well-being and aids in energy maintenance. Dehydration can result in weariness, diminished cognitive function, and poor physical performance. Individuals living with HIV/AIDS can improve their energy levels, attention, and overall quality of life by staying hydrated.

Those living with HIV/AIDS must maintain a regular schedule. Hydration can be achieved by consuming plenty of fluids throughout the day. Water is the primary and best hydration option. Herbal teas, diluted fruit juices, and clear soups are also hydrating options. However, it is critical to contact a healthcare expert to evaluate the optimum fluid consumption for each individual, as certain illnesses or drugs may necessitate changes to fluid guidelines.

To summarize, appropriate hydration is critical for HIV/AIDS management and overall health. Individuals with HIV/AIDS can support their immune system, improve medication effectiveness, promote nutritional absorption, and improve general well-being by staying hydrated.

Chapter 3

Foods To Include in an HIV/AIDS Diet

These foods supply critical nutrients, promote immunological function, and aid in overall health maintenance. Incorporating a varied range of nutrient-rich foods can contribute to better well-being in HIV/AIDS patients.

Consider the following food categories:

3.1 Fruits and vegetables

Vitamins, minerals, antioxidants, and fiber are abundant in fruits and vegetables. They supply important nutrients that help the immune system and overall wellness. Aim for a colorful assortment of leafy greens, citrus fruits, berries, cruciferous vegetables (broccoli, cauliflower), and vivid fruits such as mangoes, papayas, and tomatoes.

3.2 Whole Grains

Whole grains are an excellent source of Complex carbs, fiber, and important nutrients are all present. They provide long-lasting energy and help to maintain overall nutritional balance. Whole grain options such as whole wheat bread, brown rice, quinoa, oats, and whole grain cereals should be included.

3.3 Lean Proteins

Protein is essential for tissue repair and growth, immunological function, and muscle mass maintenance. Choose skinless poultry, fish (such as salmon, tuna, and trout), lean cuts of beef and pig, eggs, low-fat dairy products, legumes (such as lentils and chickpeas), and tofu or tempeh for plant-based protein sources.

3.4 Good Fats

It is critical to include healthy fats in your diet for overall health and nutrition absorption. Avocados, nuts (almonds, walnuts), seeds (flaxseeds, chia seeds), and olive oil are good sources of monounsaturated and polyunsaturated fats, and omega-3 fatty acid-rich fatty fish (salmon, mackerel, sardines).

3.5 Dairy or Dairy Substitutes

Calcium, protein, and vitamin D can all be found in dairy products and dairy alternatives. Choose low-fat or fat-free alternatives such as milk, yogurt, and cheese. Choose fortified dairy alternatives such as almond milk, soy milk, or oat milk if lactose intolerant or following a plant-based diet.

3.6 Nuts and legumes

Legumes like beans, lentils, and chickpeas are high in protein, fiber, and important minerals. They provide a versatile and plant-based protein source. Almonds, walnuts, and cashews are high in healthful fats, protein, and minerals. Include them in meals or serve them as snacks.

3.7 Hydration

Hydration is critical for general health and well-being. Although water is the most common source of hydration, herbal teas, diluted fruit juices, and clear soups can also help. Staying hydrated improves immunological function, assists digestion, and helps prevent dehydration-related problems.

3.8 Snacks High in Nutrients

Include nutrient-dense snacks to keep your energy levels up all day. Fresh fruits, raw veggies with hummus or yogurt-based dips, mixed nuts, seeds, Greek yogurt, or homemade energy snacks with healthful ingredients are also good choices.

3.9 Foods High in Antioxidants

Antioxidant-rich foods aid in the prevention of oxidative stress and inflammation. Berries, dark chocolate, spinach, kale, green tea, and tomatoes are abundant in antioxidants such as vitamin C, vitamin E, and phytonutrients.

Individuals can boost their vitamin intake and immune system by integrating these foods into their HIV/AIDS diet, as well as boost general wellness. Remember to consult with a trained dietitian/nutritionist for assistance.

Considerations for Nutritional Management of Symptoms and Side Effects

Proper eating can help to alleviate discomfort, maintain nutritional status, and promote general well-being. Here are some important considerations:

Nausea and Appetite Loss:

- Instead of huge meals, eat smaller, more regular meals throughout the day.
- Choose bland, easy-to-digest items such as plain crackers, rice, bread, or boiled potatoes.
- Avoid oily or fried foods, which can aggravate nausea.
- To alleviate nausea, drink clear drinks or ginger tea.

- Consider integrating anti-nausea ginger into your meals or beverages.

Diarrhea:

- Avoid foods and beverages that can cause stomach irritation. Spicy foods, high-fat foods, caffeine, and alcohol are examples.
- Include meals that are easily digestible, such as bananas, rice, applesauce, and toast (BRAT diet).
- Drink plenty of fluids, such as water, clear broths, and electrolyte-rich beverages, to stay hydrated.
- Consume soluble fiber-rich foods such as oats, cooked veggies, and peeled fruits to help bulk up stool.

Oral Thrush and Swallowing Difficulties:

- Smoothies, yogurt, pureed soups, and mashed vegetables are examples of soft, readily chewable foods.
- Avoid hot or acidic foods that may cause oral irritation.

- Hot foods may be uncomfortable, so opt for room temperature or cold items.
- Maintain good oral hygiene by brushing your teeth gently and using a light mouthwash.

Malnutrition and Weight Loss:

- To address increasing nutrient needs, prioritize the consumption of nutrient-dense meals.
- To support muscle mass, eat protein-rich meals including lean meats, fish, eggs, lentils, and dairy products.
- Increase your calorie intake by including healthy fats like avocados, almonds, and olive oil.
- Snack on calorie-dense foods such as trail mix, nut butter, and energy bars.

Consider integrating nutritional supplements or shakes as recommended by your doctor.

Tiredness and Weakness:

- Consume enough calories to keep your energy levels up.
- For prolonged energy release, include complex carbs such as whole grains, fruits, and vegetables.
- To fight fatigue caused by anemia, eat iron-rich foods such as lean red meats, spinach, beans, and fortified cereals.
- Maintain hydration to avoid dehydration, which can contribute to weariness.

Bone Wellness:

- Calcium-rich meals such as low-fat dairy products, leafy greens, and fortified plant-based milk replacements should be included. Consume vitamin D-rich foods including fatty fish (such as salmon and mackerel), egg yolks, and fortified dairy or plant-based products.

- Engage in weight-bearing workouts and consult with a healthcare practitioner about calcium and vitamin D supplementation.

Interactions Between Drugs and Nutrients:

- Certain nutrients may interact with certain HIV/AIDS drugs. To address any potential interactions, speak with a healthcare provider or a qualified dietitian.
- Discuss the usage of nutritional supplements with your healthcare physician to confirm that they are compatible with your prescriptions.
- Individuals can control symptoms and side effects linked with HIV/AIDS and its treatment by considering these nutritional measures, as well as maintaining enough nutrition and improving general well-being. It is critical to seek tailored advice from healthcare practitioners or certified dietitians based on individual needs and drug regimens.

Digestion and Nutrient Absorption Optimization

Proper digestion and nutrition absorption are critical for overall health, symptom management, and immune system support. Here are some important considerations:

Eat Mindfully: To enhance good digestion, use mindful eating strategies. Slowly and completely chew your food, appreciating each bite. Eating in a relaxing setting and focusing on the eating experience helps improve digestion by helping the body to effectively break down and absorb nutrients.

Include Foods High in Digestive Enzymes: Include foods high in digestive enzymes, such as papaya, pineapple, ginger, and fermented foods like sauerkraut or kimchi. These foods can help with macronutrient breakdown and digestion.

Consume Probiotic-Rich Foods: Probiotics are helpful microorganisms that help with digestion and support a healthy gut microbiota. Probiotic-rich foods such as yogurt, kefir, kombucha, and fermented vegetables should be included. These foods can aid with intestinal health and nutrient absorption.

Manage Stress: Chronic stress has been shown to impair digestion and nutrition absorption. Incorporate stress-management practices such as deep breathing exercises, meditation, yoga, or relaxing activities. You can support a healthy digestive system by reducing stress.

Consume a range of high-fiber foods: such as whole grains, fruits and vegetables, legumes, and nuts. Fiber encourages regular bowel movements, aids in the maintenance of a healthy gut environment, and stimulates the growth of good gut bacteria. However, if you have diarrhea, avoid high-fiber foods because they may aggravate your symptoms.

Keep Hydrated: Hydration is critical for proper digestion and nutrition absorption. Drink enough water throughout the day to help food flow through the digestive tract and maintain appropriate bowel function.

Manage Medication Side Effects: Some HIV/AIDS drugs have side effects that affect digestion. Work closely with your doctor to control these side effects and to address any digestive issues. They may be able to recommend alternate medications or supportive techniques.

Consider Nutritional Supplements: Nutritional supplements may be recommended in some circumstances to aid digestion and nutrient absorption. Digestive enzymes, probiotics, and nutritional supplements are examples of such supplements. Consult a trained dietician or a healthcare expert to decide whether supplements are required and acceptable for your unique needs.

Food Monitoring, Food Intolerances, and Allergies: Some HIV/AIDS patients may develop food intolerances or allergies. Keep an eye out for any negative reactions to certain foods and collaborate with healthcare providers to identify and treat these sensitivities. Allergy testing or elimination diets may be advised.

Individuals living with HIV/AIDS can improve their digestion, nutrient absorption, and overall health by applying these measures. Working collaboratively with healthcare specialists, particularly registered dietitians, to establish individualized plans that fit individual needs and manage any specific digestive difficulties is critical.

Meal Preparation Hints and Healthy Cooking Techniques

Proper meal preparation and cooking methods can boost the nutritional content of foods while also supporting overall wellness. Here are some important considerations:

Plan Ahead: Make a weekly meal plan to guarantee a balanced and varied diet. This will help you plan your grocery shopping and save time when preparing meals. Incorporate a variety of lean proteins, whole grains, fruits and vegetables, and healthy fats into your diet.

Select Nutritious Ingredients:

Choose nutrient-rich ingredients that add to a well-rounded diet. Choose fresh fruits and vegetables, whole grains, lean meats, and healthy fats over processed foods. To achieve a diversified nutrient profile, use a variety of hues.

Limit Processed Foods: Limit your intake of processed foods, which are frequently heavy in added sugars, harmful fats, and sodium. To enhance nutritional benefits, focus on complete, unprocessed meals.

Meal Control: Pay attention to meal sizes to maintain a well-balanced nutrient intake. To estimate proper portion sizes for different food groups, use measuring cups, a food scale, or visual cues. This can aid in weight management by preventing overeating.

Make Use of Healthy Cooking Techniques:

Choose healthy cooking methods that maintain food's nutritional value:

- Steaming: Steaming veggies helps to retain nutrients while preserving texture and color.
- Roasting/Baking: Using a tiny quantity of healthy oil to roast or bake items can improve their flavors without adding too much fat.
- Grilling provides a smokey taste to lean proteins, veggies, and fruits without the use of extra oil.
- Stir-frying: Cooking vegetables and proteins in a small amount of oil over high heat maintains their texture and nutrition.
- Boiling/Poaching: Boiling or poaching items, such as chicken, can be a healthful way to cook proteins.
- Deep frying or pan-frying with too much oil adds unneeded calories and bad fats.

Use Herbs and Spices to Add Flavor:

Experiment with herbs and spices to flavor your food without using too much salt, sugar, or unhealthy condiments. Fresh herbs like basil, cilantro, and rosemary, as well as spices like turmeric, cumin, and paprika, may give meals depth and complexity.

Reduce salt and Added Sugars: When cooking, keep salt and added sugars in mind. To enhance flavors, reduce your usage of salt and replace it with herbs, spices, citrus juice, or vinegar. Use natural sweeteners like fruits or modest amounts of honey or maple syrup to reduce added sugars.

Practice Food Safety: Ensure food safety throughout the meal, following proper cleanliness and storage measures to ensure food safety throughout meal preparation. Hands should be well washed, raw and cooked meals should be kept separate, foods should be cooked to acceptable temperatures, and leftovers should be refrigerated as soon as possible.

Meal Preparation and Batch Cooking: To save time and have healthful meals on hand, consider batch cooking and meal planning. Make larger batches of meals and split them into individual servings for later eating. This might help you stick to a balanced eating habit, even on hectic days.

Individuals with HIV/AIDS can enjoy nutritional meals that enhance their overall health and well-being by integrating these meal preparation recommendations and smart cooking techniques. Experiment with various flavors, ingredients, and cooking methods to create a varied and delightful dining experience. Remember to seek the advice of a registered nutritionist for tailored information and recommendations based on individual nutritional needs and interests.

Foods to Avoid If You Have HIV

When living with HIV, it's critical to eat a well-balanced, nutritional diet to support your immune system and general health. While no specific meals must be avoided entirely, there are some general rules to follow:

Processed and Sugary Foods: Avoid highly processed foods, sugary snacks, and sugary drinks. These can contribute to weight gain and inflammation in the body.

High-Fat Foods: While healthy fats are an important element of a balanced diet, eating too many high-fat foods, particularly those high in trans fats and saturated fats, can lead to weight gain and other health problems.

Alcohol and Recreational Drugs: Excessive alcohol intake or recreational drug use, drugs can damage the immune system, impair medicine effectiveness, and cause other health problems. If you must drink alcohol, do it in moderation.

Consumption of Raw or Undercooked Seafood and Meat: Consumption of raw or undercooked seafood, meat, and eggs may provide a risk of bacterial or parasite infection.

Unpasteurized Dairy and Cheese: Avoid unpasteurized dairy products and cheeses since they may contain hazardous bacteria.

Unwashed Fruits and Vegetables: To limit the danger of bacterial infection, always thoroughly wash fruits and vegetables.

High-Sodium Foods: Excessive salt consumption can cause high blood pressure, which may be a concern for some HIV patients. It is best to restrict your intake of high-sodium processed meals.

Grapefruit and Grapefruit Juice: Grapefruit can interfere with Some medications, especially antiretroviral treatments, are affected by the metabolism of others. Any potential interactions should be discussed with your healthcare professional.

Unregulated Herbal Supplements: Use herbal supplements with caution and contact your healthcare professional before starting any new supplements, as they can interfere with drugs or have unexpected side effects.

Individual dietary demands can vary depending on characteristics such as age, gender, exercise level, and overall health. As a result, it is strongly advised to collaborate with a healthcare physician or a certified dietitian who is educated in HIV/AIDS and nutrition. They can offer tailored advice and assist you in developing a balanced food plan that suits your specific needs and interests.

Reasons HIV Patients Should Avoid Grapefruit and Grapefruit Juice

To treat the infection and strengthen their immune system, HIV patients are frequently administered a combination of drugs known as antiretroviral therapy (ART). These drugs are critical in inhibiting HIV replication and maintaining a low viral load.

Furanocoumarins, notably bergamottin and 6',7'-dihydroxybergamottin (DHB), are found in grapefruit and grapefruit juice. These chemicals are abundant in grapefruit and can inhibit the action of certain enzymes in the liver and intestines, including cytochrome P450 enzymes CYP3A4 and CYP1A2.

Here's why this is important for people taking HIV medications:

I. **Metabolism and Absorption**: Cytochrome P450 enzymes play an important role in drug metabolism in the body. They are in charge of converting drugs into easily excretable forms. These enzymes are inhibited in the presence of grapefruit chemicals, resulting in a reduction in the metabolism of some medications.

II. **Increased Blood Levels**: When the function of these enzymes is blocked, the medicine levels in the blood can skyrocket. This may result in elevated medication levels and an increased risk of adverse effects or toxicities.

III. **Drug Effectiveness:** Increased drug levels can potentially reduce therapeutic effectiveness. For example, if the drug concentration rises above the appropriate therapeutic range, it increases the chance of unpleasant responses.

IV.   **Potential for Drug Interactions**: Many of the HIV medicines are metabolized by the same cytochrome P450 enzymes. If grapefruit components block these enzymes, it can lead to drug interactions and changes in how drugs are metabolized in the body.

Individuals may react differently to these interactions depending on their genetics, the medications they are taking, and their overall health status. Some people may be more sensitive than others to these encounters. Because of these potential interactions, healthcare providers often advise HIV patients to avoid grapefruit and grapefruit juice. Other citrus fruits, such as oranges and lemons, do not contain the same chemicals and are therefore safe to consume.

If you have any questions or concerns, always consult your healthcare professional or pharmacist about potential drug-drug interactions with specific foods or beverages. They can give you individualized advice based on your drugs and health situation.

What should an HIV patient do if he or she mistakenly takes something that slows metabolism?

If an HIV patient inadvertently consumes food that may impair metabolism or interfere with drug absorption, it is critical to take preventative measures.

What you can do is as follows:

Remain Calm: First and foremost, try to remain cool. Accidents occur, and it is critical not to panic.

Identify the Causing Factor: If possible, pinpoint the exact meal or item that may be interfering with metabolism or drug absorption. This will aid in determining the potential impact.

Contact the following healthcare provider: As soon as possible, contact the patient's healthcare physician or pharmacist. They are most suited to provide tailored advice based on the patient's exact drug regimen and health situation.

Provide Specifics: When calling the healthcare professional, be careful to include detailed data about what was consumed, such as the sort of food or substance consumed, the amount consumed, and the time it was consumed.

Follow Professional Advice: Follow the advice of your healthcare provider. They may advise specific activities based on the circumstances. This could include any changes to medication dosages or regimens that are required.

Observe for Symptoms: Keep a watch out for any unexpected symptoms or side effects. If there are any apparent changes in how the patient feels, notify the healthcare professional right away.

Maintain Hydration: Remind the patient to stay hydrated. Proper hydration is essential for general health and can help the body digest chemicals.

Avoiding Additional Consumption: Ensure that the patient refrains from consuming the problematic food or drug until they receive advice from their healthcare physician.

Use the incident to educate both the patient and any caregivers about foods or substances that may interact with their prescriptions. This can aid in the prevention of such events in the future.

Remember that in instances like this, it's critical to talk with a healthcare expert. They know to provide tailored advice based on the medications the patient is taking, their overall health, and the nature of the interaction.

Additionally, always follow up with the healthcare practitioner following the occurrence to discuss any concerns or issues that may have arisen. They can provide continuing assistance and ensure that the patient's needs are met.

Conclusion

We examined different elements of nutrition for people living with HIV/AIDS in this detailed guide. Understanding the unique challenges and nutritional requirements connected with this illness allows us to make informed decisions that benefit our overall health and well-being.

We have discussed the need to seek expert advice and the role of medical considerations in managing HIV/AIDS nutrition, from knowing the basics of HIV/AIDS to negotiating the intricate link between nutrition and immune function. We've also talked about necessary nutrients for immune support, how to create balanced meal plans, portion control, mindful eating, and the importance of hydration in HIV/AIDS management.

Furthermore, we investigated items to include in an HIV/AIDS diet, strategies for managing symptoms and negative effects, and strategies for enhancing digestion and nutrient absorption, as well as meal planning advice and healthy cooking practices. Individuals can optimize their nutrition, increase their immune function, manage symptoms and side effects, and improve their general quality of life by adopting these recommendations into their everyday lives.

It is critical to remember that each person's HIV/AIDS journey is unique, and personalized counsel from healthcare professionals, particularly registered dietitians, is crucial. They can make unique recommendations based on your needs, medications, and medical conditions.

Individuals living with HIV/AIDS can take an active role in controlling their health and supporting their immune system by combining medical treatment, adherence to antiretroviral medicine, and a well-balanced, nutritional diet.

Remember that this book is only a beginning point, providing information and ideas to help people become more self-sufficient. Individuals can negotiate the obstacles of HIV/AIDS with resilience and lead full lives by adopting a holistic approach to health.

Let us continue to encourage and support one another while recognizing the importance of nutrition as a crucial component of comprehensive HIV/AIDS care. We can create a community that lives on knowledge, compassion, and perseverance in the face of hardship if we work together.

I wish you good health, happiness, and a bright future.